Ketogenic Vegetarian

TABLE OF CONTENTS

INTRODUCTION 4
CHAPTER ONE: WHAT IS KETOGENIC VEGETARIAN DIET 6
CHAPTER TWO: KETOSIS IS NOT KETOACIDOSIS 11
CHAPTER THREE: IS A KETOGENIC DIET FOR VEGETARIANS REASONABLY POSSIBLE? 17
    VEGETARIAN KETO CLUB SALAD 26
    NOATMEAL 27
    KETO OVERNIGHT "OATS" 28
    CHIA SEED PUDDING RECIPE 29
    CINNAMON KETO GRANOLA 30
    CINNAMON FRENCH TOFU STICKS WITH CHOCOLATE SYRUP 31
    VEGAN KETO SANDWICH BREAD 33
    BASIC VEGAN FRENCH TOAST 34
    VEGAN FRENCH TOAST 35
    GLUTEN FREE VEGAN KETO BAGELS 36
    AVOCADO SPREAD 37
    HOMEMADE SAMBAL 38
    VEGAN SESAME TOFU AND EGGPLANT 39
    ZUCCHINI RIBBONS & AVOCADO WALNUT PESTO 41
    LOW CARB FRIED MAC & CHEESE 43
    TOMATO BASIL AND MOZZARELLA GALETTE 44
    KETO GRILLED CHEESE SANDWICH 46
    FRESH BELL PEPPER BASIL PIZZA 47
    KETO BREAKFAST BROWNIE MUFFINS 49
    VEGETARIAN GREEK COLLARD WRAPS 50
    SUN DRIED TOMATO PESTO MUG CAKE 52
    SESAME ALMOND ZOODLE BOWL 53
    CHEESY THYME WAFFLES 55
    CHEESY HEARTS OF PALM DIP 56
    LOW CARB BROCCOLI AND CHEESE FRITTERS 57
    WARM ASIAN BROCCOLI SALAD 59
    CAULIFLOWER MAC & CHEESE 60
    PERSONAL PAN PIZZA DIP 61
    VEGETARIAN THREE CHEESE QUICHE STUFFED PEPPERS 63

- ROASTED MUSHROOM AND WALNUT CAULIFLOWER GRITS 64
- CHARRED VEGGIE AND FRIED GOAT CHEESE SALAD 66
- CRISPY TOFU AND BOK CHOY SALAD 67
- VEGETARIAN GREEK COLLARD WRAPS 69
- SESAME ALMOND ZOODLE BOWL 71
- VEGETARIAN THREE CHEESE QUICHE STUFFED PEPPERS 73
- VEGETARIAN RED COCONUT CURRY 74
- VEGAN KETO PORRIDGE 75
- LEMON RASPBERRY SWEET ROLLS 76
- KETO BREAKFAST BROWNIE MUFFINS 80
- AVOCADO CHOCOLATE MOUSSE 81
- CAULIFLOWER SOUP 83
- CHEESY EGG MUFFINS 84
- ITALIAN BAKED EGG AND VEGETABLES 85
- KETO TABBOULEH 86
- VEGAN KETO COOKIE CARAMEL COOKIE BARS 87
- KETO COCONUT DULCE DE LECHE 89
- VEGAN KETO MAPLE CINNAMON NOATMEAL 90
- PANCAKE MUFFINS 91
- POPPY SEED MUFFINS 92
- PIZZA BREAKFAST FRITTATA 93
- MOCK MCGRIDDLE LOAF 94
- CAULIFLOWER AND JALAPENO CHEESE 95
- KETO FRIENDLY SUSHI 97
- CHOCOLATE AND COCONUT BARS 98
- CHOCOLATE MUG CAKE 99
- CHOCOLATE AND PEANUT BUTTER TARTS 100
- VEGAN POTATO NACHOS 102
- MUSHROOM AND KALE ENCHILADAS WITH RED SAUCE 104
- ENCHILADAS 106
- SUPER EASY VEGGIE MAC AND CHEESE 108
- WARM GREEN BEANS AND LETTUCE IN ANCHOVY BUTTER .. 109
- CONCLUSION 110

INTRODUCTION

A ketogenic diet is one that requires us to reduce the number of calories we eat to below the amount of calories our bodies use in a day, triggering the release of energy that is stored as fat in our body's cells. This fat is also called ketones, which our muscles use as fuel. Of course, there is a big difference between starving yourself and simply reducing your caloric intake in a way that keeps you satisfied and healthy.

This book illustrates the idea that long term success at maintaining fat loss requires that we feel good during and after weight loss. Maintaining steady energy levels, keeping your moods stable, and the fun and excitement of creating your own desired changes are the keys to your success.

This type of ketogenic diet does not mean over-eating huge slabs of meat. Likewise, it does it mean over-indulging in fried or fatty foods or completely eliminating carbohydrates.

Some people have misused the idea of low-carb ketogenic diets by misinterpreting the intention of clinicians who promote this method. As a result, the media as well as some medical authorities have emphasize the "dangers" or "failures" that have followed the extreme behaviors adopted by some people. In fact, this book overwhelmingly shows that a low-carb ketogenic diet is not only safe, but is also effective for fat loss.

As you read, you will also learn more about the following...

- Delicious and healthy recipes for rapid weight loss
- What a Ketogenic Vegetarian Diet is
- Why we should follow a Ketogenic Vegetarian Diet
- Delicious and easy Ketogenic Vegetarian recipes
- How we eat to lose weight
- Ketosis is not a ketoacidosis
- Whether or not a Vegetarian Ketogenic Diet is possible
- Recommended and advisable foods
- Fat for vegetarians in ketosis
- Protein sources on a Vegetarians Ketogenic Diet

Using this book is best for you and your family.

CHAPTER ONE

WHAT IS KETOGENIC VEGETARIAN DIET

Not everyone with PCOS is obviously overweight, however, the health of everyone with PCOS is threatened by the body chemistry that results from eating either a standard America diet, or a standard vegetarian diet.

PCOS is a version of what is also known as Metabolic Syndrome, or Syndrome X. This is the condition that results in men, women, and (sadly) in more and more children in recent years. This condition is a result of overeating foods that are highly processed, artificially flavored and preserved, high refined flour and full of simple carbohydrates.

The excess of sweets, breads, pastas, cereals, and packaged foods provides many more calories than the average person uses in a day. Even organically grown grains, eaten whole or manufactured into "wholesome" forms of old favorites like chips, cookies, etc., will have the same effect as excess sugar when over eaten. The insulin required to process all the blood sugar that results from diets that are high in sugar, flour, etc., is what causes higher levels of testosterone in women.

Increased levels of testosterone can then lead to hormone imbalances which cause polycystic ovaries, infertility, acne, facial hair, and hair thinning. Left unchanged, this diet caneventually cause obesity, diabetes, and heart disease; it creates a higher risk for certain cancers as well.

Foods high in carbohydrates can lead to:
- Elevated insulin levels
- Elevated testosterone levels
- Menstrual disorders
- Facial and body hair darkening and becoming coarse
- Hair thinning on the scalp
- Acne
- Increased risk for infertility, obesity, diabetes, heart disease, and certain cancers

Once you have extra fat, you have to eat in a special way for what I call a "therapeutic interval". This simply means that there are certain changes that you have to make and a certain amount of time is required for fat loss to be fully successful. This special way of eating does not have to be the way you will eat the rest of your life... IF you include building muscle and using your muscle while losing this fat. The more muscle you have, the more calories you must consume to be healthy. Similarly, with little muscle and not much exercise, there is not much you can eat without your body storing fat.

How We Eat to Lose Weight
The most reliable and straightforward way to use up stored fat is through a diet that eliminates unnecessary sweets and starchy carbohydrates while also providing

plenty of fresh, whole vegetables, fruit, nuts, good quality oils and lean, clean animal protein.

Almost every successful weight loss diet is a ketogenic diet. A ketogenic diet is where we reduce our total caloric intake to below the amount of calories our bodies use in a day, triggering the release of energy stored as fat in our body cells. This fat is in the form of chemistry called ketones, which our muscles use as fuel. Of course, there is a big difference between starving yourself and reducing your calories in a way that keeps you satisfied and healthy!

Ultimately our long term success at maintaining fat loss requires that we feel good during and after weight loss. Maintaining steady energy levels, keeping your moods stable, and the fun and excitement of creating your own desired changes are the keys to your success.

It turns out that you can burn more fat while eating a larger number of calories when you get fewer of your calories from carbohydrates and more from good, quality protein and fat. This type of ketogenic diet does not mean over-eating huge slabs of meat. Likewise, it does not mean over-indulging in fried or fatty foods or completely eliminating carbohydrates.

Some people have misused the idea of low-carb ketogenic diets by misinterpreting the intention of clinicians who promote this method. As a result, the media as well as some medical authorities have emphasize the "dangers" or "failures" that have followed the extreme behaviors adopted by some people. In fact, this book overwhelmingly shows that a low-carb ketogenic diet is not only safe, but is also effective for fat loss.

Remember, we can only lose fat by reducing our caloric intake to less than the amount of calories we use in our daily activities. This is a fundamental truth. However, there are many additional details that make this strategy more or less likely to succeed, especially over time. Some conditions that complicate the basic calories-fat-reduced equation include:

 * Chronic stress that fatigues your adrenal function
* Chronic pain that keeps your nervous system on high alert
* Insomnia that reduces the opportunity for your organs to perform restorative functions that will not happen except during deep sleep
* Perimenopause or other conditions that alter your reproductive hormone functions (including the use of contraceptive hormones, hormone replacement therapy, a hysterectomy, and breastfeeding)
* Thyroid disorders
* Kidney disease
* Any immobilizing condition

All of these conditions can be addressed with a diet plan as well as a transition plan that is personalized to your situation.

One important detail to our weight loss success has to do with how we feel physically, mentally, and emotionally when we reduce calories. If we simply eat less without regarding the composition of our diet, i.e., the fat, protein, and carbohydrate content as well as the vitamins and minerals that we need, chances are that we will have an unpleasant experience. This is because hunger, fatigue, headaches, muscle spasms, mental fogginess, depression, irritability, and insomnia are common experiences shared by dieters who use low fat, low calorie, high carbohydrate diets. With these diets, we can also find ourselves losing weight that includes muscle mass along with fat we wanted to lose.

In a low-carb ketogenic diet, we reduce our calories from starchy carbohydrates in particular and nourish our selves with appropriate amounts of water, vegetables, fruit, eggs, poultry, fish, meat, nuts, and good quality oils. This change helps to creates fat loss without the usual unpleasant side effects. It also helps us to identify problem foods, so that when we transition from a fat loss diet to a more "natural" diet to maintain weight, we can do so without returning to old food-related problems.

CHAPTER TWO

KETOSIS IS NOT KETOACIDOSIS

Ketones are a product of fat metabolism and function as a source of energy for the body. Our muscles as well as other tissues can use ketones for fuel instead of glucose, or blood sugar. Ketones are released from stored fat and then used for energy when there is not enough glucose available. This is because our brains require blood sugar for fuel whereas muscles and other metabolic processes can take up ketones instead. Additionally, we can make blood glucose from everything we eat, including by transforming proteins from animal foods. We can not, however, make protein for our bodies from plant foods. Rather, what we end up making from the carbohydrates of plant food is fat. The excess carbohydrates we eat every day beyond what we use when exercising our muscles is transformed into and stored as fat. This was a great system for people (like our human ancestors) who do not have a reliable food supply and are subject to regular periods of feast or famine. For most of us, however, it means that we have an ever enlarging "storage bin" of accumulated fat.

There is some confusion regarding the ketosis that occurs when we are eating fewer carbohydrates than we need for daily fuel and begin to burn stored fat instead. Some people confuse normal, beneficial ketosis with something known as ketoacidosis which occurs when people with high blood sugar levels i.e., diabetics, simultaneously produce high levels of ketones.

People with diabetes do not produce enough insulin from their pancreas, or they have a condition called insulin resistance which is when tissues no longer respond to the presence of insulin bearing glucose that is being delivered into storage. Ketones are formed in response to the tissues need for some fuel other than the glucose, which is collecting in the blood attached to insulin molecules but can no longer be delivered into cells. Generally, our bodies will adjust the blood pH level to balance this shifting chemistry; however, in diabetics, the imbalance is too great causing ketoacidosis, or increased acidity of the blood to occur. Metabolic ketoacidosis in people with diabetes is a dangerous condition and should be avoided with very strict control and attention to diet as well as blood sugar levels.

When a person with normal blood sugar levels produces ketones by breaking down fat for fuel while not eating excess carbohydrates, blood glucose is delivered elegantly, primarily to the brain, and the rest of the body happily uses ketones to run the show.

Eating foods that are rich in carbohydrates in amounts that allow for the release of ketones from stored fat is a safe and effective way to reduce body fat while maintaining an even blood sugar levels. Keeping your blood sugar levels stable means you will have plenty of physical energy, be mentally alert, and experience restful sleep. Most people can eat this way for the rest of their lives and be quite well, and most people will actually want to diversify their diet after having lost excess fat. Expanding your diet to include more fruits, grains, and appropriate celebratory treats can be accomplished without regaining fat.

This transition has to be done thoughtfully and with close attention to the impact of certain foods. For example, some people will never be able to eat certain foods without experienceing negative consequences because of their genetic make up. Regardless, we all have to reintroduce foods carefully and maintain exercise throughout our lives in order not to regain lost fat.

A ketogenic fat loss diet is not appropriate for pregnancy and breastfeeding as these are times when fat stores are very important to the wellbeing of both the mother and her baby/babies. Additionally, people with kidney damage, diabetes, epilepsy, and gall bladder problems should not use this diet unless they will be closely supervised by their physician.

Women lose weight somewhat slower than men because feminine hormones, i.e., estrogen, effects how women hold onto water and fat. In general, men have greater muscle mass, even when quite fat. In addition to hormones such as testosterone, this help them burn fat somewhat more effectively than women. Regardless, regular exercise is absolutely necessary for everyone's long term health.

How we transition from fat loss to long term healthy diet determines our long term success.

Transitioning successfully from a fat loss diet to a healthy life long diet is only beginning to be understood. Specifics for success include:

* A metabolic readjustment period (5 to 10 or more weeks)
* Educational support that works with the habits of thought and feelings surrounding body image and our learned eating and exercise behaviors.

Whenever we let go of stored energy (a.k.a. fat) by reducing our caloric intake, primitive protective mechanisms in our brains kick in and our basic metabolic rate starts to slow down. When this happens, our bodies actually start using less fat to protect us from what our ancestrial hard-wired brain thinks is a famine. For our human ancestors, an unreliable food supply made this trait essential for survival. For those of us who are eating less by choice, however, this mechanism is what will cause us to regain weight we have lost as soon as we start eating "normally" again.

That "normal" eating concept is key. If you get fat, then you need to eat to lose fat, but when you have reached your goal weight, you resume eating the way you did that got you fat in the first place and the cycle continues like that. Not only are you eating the same food that caused you to gain weight again, you are piling it into a body that is newly programmed to burn less energy during your regular daily activities. In some cases, you may also have have lost muscle mass. In order to complete the change to a forever-leaner you, fat loss is truly only step one.

Step two is working to re-set your metabolic rate to where is was or higher than it was before you began your fat loss diet. How that is done is a mystery that has frustrated the many dieters; it has also caused a great deal of unhealthy and frustrating yo-yo patterns of weight loss and regain.

We know that 90% of people who lose weight regain what they lost and then some. However, some people do not regain weight and recent research has examined what is different about this fascinating 10%. Essentially what these folks do differently is they become acutely aware of small amounts weight regained, and they return to their weight loss behaviors for brief periods of time to lose what they have regained. Eventually, as long as they maintain consistently healthy habits, including their food choices and exercise levels, the episodes of weight gain stop and they stabilize at their new weight.

Transitioning to healthy eating after losing weight requires:
* Having an established, regular, and fun exercise habit once you arrive at your goal weight
* Keeping very close tabs on your weight as well as on your inches at your waist and hips
* Returning to weight loss behaviors whenever you have regained 2 to 3 pounds.
* After returning to weight loss behaviors, expand your food choices again until you eventually stabilize at yous goal weight with your new commitment to and enjoyment of regular exercise.
* Continue maintaining a healthy muscle mass, activity level, and consistently adjust your diet to one that consists of fresh, whole foods as you age and/or encounter new circumstances or health challenges

Remember – there is one proven way that we need to eat to lose fat, and another more generous and complex way we can eat once our goal is attained. The nature of the transition between these two ways of eating is essential to long term success. However, the ability to lose weight, make dietary changes that are less stringent and more varied, then return as often as needed to the weight loss regime for brief periods until stabilized, is apparently a rare ability. Most people do not seem to discover this behavior spontaneously. Thus, long term guidance and support is crucial.

A number of studies on successful weight loss have clarified that knowledgeable support helps people to not only remember the basic, straightforward steps of the diet cha-cha, but also helps them expand their skills for stress management, exercise options, and cooking skills. Often times, the benefits and habits that are leaned during this process benefit everyone around you, including your family.

We have many behaviors and beliefs that affect our sense of self and our ability to pursue long-term self-discipline. It is clear that ongoing and specific support, in the form of individual counseling or a similar support group experience, makes success much more likely. We encourage you to use both the weight loss and maintenance aspects of the program described here, while also adding in regular exercise and regular contact with a knowledgeable and/or skilled support system to ensure long term results.

CHAPTER THREE

IS A KETOGENIC DIET FOR VEGETARIANS REASONABLY POSSIBLE?

Regardless of your motives for cutting out animal meat, you are probably equally aware of all the buzz about the ketogenic diet and wondering if you can go keto while staying away from all meats.

The answer is "yes", but it takes a little extra thought. While the traditional keto diet typically involves a lot of meat for protein, it's not necessary to eat meat while following the plan. In fact, the biggest component of the ketogenic diet is good fat, which you can easily get from vegetarian foods.

For omnivores going keto, the most common mistake is eating too much protein.

Similarly, the biggest mistake that vegetarians make whengoing keto is eating too many carbohydrates from vegetables. You do have to be a little more careful with your carb and protein choices since traditional vegetarian forms of protein include things like beans and grains, which aren't a part of a keto diet.

Let's tackle this by discussing the three macronutrients one at a time.

Carbohydrates for a Vegetarian Ketogenic Diet

Since vegetarian diets are typically higher in carbs than carnivorous diets, it's especially important to understand the "right" types of carbs when following a vegetarian2 ketogenic diet.

Good Carbs vs. Bad Carbs

Besides getting plenty of healthy fats, watching your carb intake is one of the most important factors here—and many go-to meals, especially snacks common for vegetarians and vegans, are pretty carb-heavy. However, to reiterate, excessive carbohydrates (even from veggies) aren't part of a keto diet and ff course, refined carbs like sugar, flour, bread, cereal, chips, etc. are immediately off the table.

Bad Carbs (High Glycemic; Highly Processed)

Here are some carb sources to remove from your home and kitchen:

- Pastas
- Breads
- Chips, crackers, and pretzels
- Tortillas
- Rice
- Sodas
- Cereals
- Packaged foods with refined sugars or flours
- Fruit juices and most fruits
- White potatoes and sweet potatoes
- Starchy vegetables

Good carbs on a vegetarian keto diet are basically the same as those on a normal keto diet including low-carb fruits, full-fat yogurts, and low-carb veggies.

Good Carbs (Limited) for a Vegetarian on Keto

Low-carb Vegetables

If you're one of those vegetarians who hates vegetables, this diet is going to be harder for you. While the most important aspect of keto is keeping your fat content high, you'll need healthy low-carb veggies to provide enough bulk and fiber to fill in your meals and get enough to eat.

Don't be afraid to explore and open yourself up to trying new vegetables in different ways. For instance, if raw veggies turn you off, try cooking some in coconut oil or butter with herbs and/or seasonings. Give yourself time to get used to the changes. Here are some low-carb vegetables to rely on:

- Spinach
- Kale
- Collard greens
- Swiss chard
- Lettuce
- Asparagus
- Green beans
- Broccoli
- Cucumber
- Summer and winter squash
- Red and white cabbage
- Cauliflower

- Bell peppers
- Onions
- Mushrooms
- Tomatoes
- Eggplants
- Garlic

Fruits

As a general rule, all fruits should be limited, however, berries are lower in sugars and carbs so they're typically okay in small amounts and at the end of the day before you fast while sleeping:

- Blackberries
- Strawberries
- Raspberries
- Blueberries

Non-Carbs to Mention (Condiments and Spices)

Spices

- Basil
- Oregano
- Parsley
- Rosemary
- Thyme
- Cilantro
- Cayenne pepper

- Chili powder
- Cumin
- Cinnamon
- Nutmeg
- Lemon or lime juice
- Pepper and salt

Protein on a Vegetarian Ketogenic Diet

Here's a comprehensive list of foods which contain protein that have the green light on a keto vegetarian diet:
Vegetarian Ketogenic Proteins

- Eggs
- Dairy
- Tempeh
- Natto
- Miso
- Nuts and seeds (see below)

If you do choose to eat soy products at all, try to stick to only those that are non-GMO and fermented (like organic tempeh).

If you find your protein needs still aren't being met, consider using an organic rice or hemp protein powder, but only use it as a supplement and not a regular meal replacement. Additionally, just remember that getting too much protein is a common ketogenic diet mistake that prevents your body from entering ketosis.

Be wary of packaged vegan and vegetarian meat substitutes, for while these might be good substitutes for meat in terms of fat and protein, they might also contain a high amount of carbs. Be sure to check the ingradients as well as the carb content per serving. Is it full or preservatives and fillers? If so, better meat substitutes would be any of the proteins mentioned above as well as portobello mushrooms or eggplant.

Fats for Vegetarians in Ketosis
Nuts and Seeds

Nuts and seeds are great sources of protein and fat, just be sure to choose mostly low-carb and high-fat choices because some nuts and seeds are higher in carbs than others and can add up quickly. Check out our full guide to nuts on the ketogenic diet and recipes like our insanely easy Macadamia Nut Fat Bomb.
Best nut options (low carb):
- Pecans
- Brazil nuts
- Macadamia nuts
- Walnuts
- Coconut (unsweetened)
- Hazelnuts
- Pine nuts
- Almonds
- Nut butters made from any of the above

Ketogenic Diet for Vegetarians

Nut options to eat sparingly or not at all (high carb):

- Peanuts
- Pistachios
- Cashews
- Chestnuts

Best seed options:

- Chia seeds
- Flaxseeds

Healthy Oils

The right types of oils are great for a ketogenic diet because they're entirely made of fat. MCT's in particular are a type of fat that metabolizes quicker than most and then broken down into useable energy. It also can easily cross the blood-brain barrier, which is why they are so beneficial to our mental clarity and performance. Here are some more great options:

- Olive oil
- Coconut oil
- Avocado oil
- MCT oil
- Macadamia oil
- Flaxseed oil

Other Non-Dairy Fat Sources
- Olives
- Avocados
- Cocoa butter
- Coconut cream

Dairy and Eggs
- Heavy whipping cream
- Cream cheese
- Cottage cheese
- Mayonnaise
- Hard cheeses like parmesan, swiss, feta, and cheddar (full-fat)
- Soft cheese like brie, Monterrey jack, mozzarella, and bleu cheese (full-fat)
- Butter (grass-fed)
- Eggs (pastured or free-range and preferably omega-3-enriched)
- Full-fat unsweetened Greek yogurt or coconut yogurt

Breakfasts Ideas
- Vegetables and eggs with avocado fried in coconut or olive oil
- Egg frittata with asparagus and avocado
- Vegetable and feta omelet fried in coconut or olive oil
- Smoothie made from coconut cream, berries, ice, full-fat yogurt, almond butter, and stevia extract

Lunch Ideas
- Egg and avocado salad
- Mixed greens salad with avocado, mozzarella, pesto, olives, bell pepper, onions, nuts, lemon juice, and extra virgin olive oil dressing
- Vegetarian low-carb Greek salad with feta, tomatoes, onions, olives, fresh Greek spices, and extra virgin olive oil
- Stir-fried cauliflower "rice" with veggies and eggs

Dinner Ideas
- Cheese pizza with cauliflower crust and broccoli

VEGETARIAN KETO CLUB SALAD

Ingredient

2 tbsp sour cream
2 tbsp mayonnaise
1/2 tsp garlic powder
1/2 tsp onion powder
1 tsp dried parsley
1 tbsp milk
3 large hard boiled eggs, sliced
4 ounces cheddar cheese, cubed
3 cups romaine lettuce, torn into pieces
1/2 cup cherry tomatoes, halved
1 cup diced cucumber
1 tbsp dijon mustard

Directions

Prepare the dressing by mixing the sour cream, mayonnaise, and dried herbs until combined.

Add one tbsp of milk and mix. If the dressing seems too thick, feel free to add another tbsp of milk but don't forget to add another tbsp of milk to the final fat/protein/carb count if you do!

Layer your salad with the fresh veggies, cheese, and sliced egg. Add a spoonful of Dijon mustard in the center.

Drizzle with the prepared dressing, about 2 tbsp for one serving, then toss to coat.

NOATMEAL

Ingredients
1/2 cup (120 ml) water (see Note)
2 tbsp hemp hearts
2 tbsp almond flour
2 tbsp unsweetened shredded coconut
1 tbsp flaxseed meal
1 tbsp chia seeds
1/4 tsp granulated stevia (or any kind of sweetener you like to taste)
1 pinch sea salt
1/2 tsp pure vanilla extract

Directions
Stove top *Directions* Add all ingredients except for the vanilla to a small saucepan over low heat. Cook until thickened, stirring constantly, about 3 to 5 minutes. Stir in the vanilla and serve warm.
Microwave *Directions* Add all ingredients except for the vanilla to a large cereal bowl that's microwave-safe. Microwave on high until thickened, about 2 minutes. Stir in the vanilla and serve warm.

KETO OVERNIGHT "OATS"

Ingredients
Vanilla Keto Overnight Oats
⅔ cup (160 ml) full-fat coconut milk (plus more for the following day)
1/2 cup (75 grams) Manitoba Harvest Hemp Hearts
1 tbsp chia seed
2 tsps confectioners' erythritol or 3 to 4 drops of liquid stevia
1/2 tsp vanilla extract
A pinch of finely ground Himalayan rock salt
Optional Toppings
12 whole almonds, omit for nut-free
6 whole raspberries

Directions
Add all ingredients to a 12 fl. oz. (350 ml), or larger container with a lid and stir until combined. Cover and set in the fridge overnight, for at least 8 hours.
The following day, add additional milk until desired consistency is reached.
Divide between two small bowls, add toppings if desired.

CHIA SEED PUDDING RECIPE

Ingredients
2 cups coconut milk (homemade or natural)
1/2 cup Chia Seeds
1/2 tsp vanilla extract
1/4 cup (or less) maple syrup (or sub any sweetener)
Optional: 1/4 tsp cinnamon powder

Directions
For Blended/Smooth Version: Place all ingredients in a blender and blend on high for 1-2 minutes until completely smooth.

For Whole Chia Seed Version: Blend all ingredients except chia seeds in a blender until smooth (including any added flavors, fruits, or chocolate). After everything is blended, whisk in the chia seeds.

Pour mixture into a jar or glass container and place in the refrigerator for at least 4 hours or overnight to let gel. Within the first hour, be sure to stir or whisk t fhe mixture a few times to help it gel evenly. I recommend making this at night to have ready for a quick breakfast the next day. It is also great to make in the morning for a delicious pre-made dessert at night.

CINNAMON KETO GRANOLA

Ingredients
5 tbsp ground flax meal
5 tbsp unsweetened coconut flakes
1 tbsp Chia Seeds
1.5 oz nuts (we used pecans, walnuts and almonds)
4 tbsp sugar free maple syrup
1 1/2 tsp Cinnamon Optional

Directions
Thoroughly combine all ingredients except for the cinnamon.
Spread mixture onto a baking sheet, making one even layer.
Sprinkle cinnamon on top.
Bake at 350 degrees for 20-22 minutes.
Let rest. Granola will harden as it cools. Enjoy!

CINNAMON FRENCH TOFU STICKS WITH CHOCOLATE SYRUP

Ingredients
1 block extra firm tofu
4 tbsp Lakanto Monk Fruit Sweetener
1 tbsp cinnamon

For the chocolate syrup:
1/2 tbsp meted coconut oil
1 tbsp cacao or cocoa powder
Lakanto Maple-Flavored Syrup to taste

Directions
1. Drain tofu and wrap it in paper towels for 10-15 minutes.
2. While the tofu is draining, combine cinnamon and Lakanto in a mixing bowl for the cinnamon-sugar topping.
3. When the tofu is done draining, cut into uniform sticks and sprinkle with 1/4 of the cinnamon-sugar topping.
4. Spray frypan with cooking spray on low heat. Place the tofu in pan.
5. Flip tofu every 3-4 minutes for about 30 minutes or until it is firm to the touch. Sprinkle tofu with more of the cinnamon-sugar topping after each flip until you've used all of the topping.
6. When the tofu is finished, prepare chocolate syrup.
7. Heat coconut oil in microwave for 30 seconds or until it liquifies.

8. Add cacao powder and liquid stevia to the coconut oil and mix thoroughly.
9. Drizzle chocolate syrup over the tofu sticks.

VEGAN KETO SANDWICH BREAD

Ingredients
160 g chia seeds
2 1/4 tsp instant yeast or one packet
800 mL warm water
100 g tahini or almond butter
100 g psyllium husks
10 g xanthan gum or guar gum
300 g almond flour
2 tsp salt
vegan keto bread 2

Directions
Mix the tahini and water together followed by the yeast and chia. Let sit for 20 mins or so until the chia is ready.

Mix the almond flour, psyllium husks, and gum with the salt.

When the chia mix is nice and goopy, mix it into your dry ingredients, kneading it until it comes together. Grease or line you bread tin with some parchment.

Add dough to tin and let rise in a warm place for at least an hour.

Bake in a 325 degrees oven for 90-120 mins until the internal temp reaches 200 degrees.

BASIC VEGAN FRENCH TOAST

Ingredients
1 heaping Tbsp chia seeds (whole or ground into a fine meal so that they're undetectable)
1/2 Tbsp agave nectar or maple syrup
1 cup unsweetened almond milk (or any non-dairy milk)
1/2 tsp ground cinnamon
1/2 tsp vanilla extract
4-5 bread slices (it's important to use a sturdy, rustic bread or it can turn out soggy/soft)

Directions
Mix all ingredients except the bread in a large, shallow bowl. Place in the fridge to marinade for 10-20 minutes.
Preheat griddle to medium heat (~350 degrees F / 176 C) and grease with 1 tbsp vegan butter or coconut oil.
Dip each slice of bread in the batter for about 20 seconds on each side. If your bread is dry, leave it in a little longer. Similarly, if you're using sandwich bread, it should only need 25-30 seconds total to soak.
Cook on a griddle until golden brown on the underside. Carefully flip and cook until the other side is golden brown as well, about 3-4 minutes.
Top with desired toppings such as coconut whipped cream, strawberries, and maple syrup.

VEGAN FRENCH TOAST

Ingredients
6 slices bread
1 cup non-dairy milk
2 tbsp silken tofu
1 tbsp nutritional yeast
1 tbsp sucanat or brown sugar
1 tsp vanilla
1/2 tsp sea salt
1/2 tsp cinnamon
dash of nutmeg

Directions
Put all ingredients except for the bread into a blender and blend until smooth. Preheat a skillet with oil, making sure to use a non-stick pan.
Dip the bread slices into the blended mixture and then place onto the skillet. Cook on both sides until browned. Serve with fruit and pure maple syrup if desired. Serves 2-3.

GLUTEN FREE VEGAN KETO BAGELS

Ingredients
3 tbsp flax seeds I used golden
1/2 cup tahini
1/4 cup psyllium powder
1/4 cup almond flour
1 tsp baking powder
1 cup water

Directions
Grind the flax seeds and add to psyllium, almond flour, and baking powder. You can choose to add salt here too if desired.
Mix water and tahini until smooth and then add to dry mix. Then, mix well until it is all combined, forming a dough ball.
Break into four pieces and shape into buns. You can either stick your finger though to make a hole like I do, or you can use a cutter.
Bake at 375 degrees for 45 mins.
When you're ready to serve, cut in half and re-toast for best texture.

AVOCADO SPREAD

Ingredients
2 medium ripe avocados
2 Tbsp fresh coriander leaves (finely chopped)
1 Tbsp fresh parsley leaves (finely chopped)
1/2 Tbsp fresh mint leaves (finely chopped)
1 garlic clove (crushed)
1/4 tsp ground cumin
juice of 1 to 2 lemons
1 roasted pepper (from a jar) finely chopped
sprinkle sunflower seeds
salt& pepper

Directions
Halve the avocados, scoop them out, and mash with a fork.
Add crushed garlic, ground cumin, chopped herbs, lemon juice, and roasted peppers.
Mixed together. Season to taste.
Spread on your favourite bread or bagel and sprinkle with sunflower seeds.

HOMEMADE SAMBAL

Ingredient
1 large onion
0.35 ounces dried birds-eye chilis
3 tbsp reduced sugar ketchup
2 tbsp coconut oil
1/2 tsp salt (or to taste)
Optional: 1-2 drops liquid sucralose

Directions
Chop onion and blend until smooth. Set aside.
Cut dried chilis and remove seeds. Boil them for about 30 minutes or until they are soft. Once soft and cooled, blend them to form a paste.
In a heated pan, melt coconut oil. Once hot, add the remaining ingredients. Optional: add in 1-2 drops Liquid Sucralose.

VEGAN SESAME TOFU AND EGGPLANT

Ingredient
1 pound block of firm tofu
1 cup (31g) chopped cilantro
3 tbsp rice vinegar
4 tbsp toasted sesame oil
2 cloves garlic, finely minced
1 tsp crushed red pepper flakes
2 tsps Swerve confectioners
1 whole (458 g) eggplant
1 tbsp olive oil
Salt and pepper to taste
1/4 cup sesame seeds
1/4 cup soy sauce

Directions
Preheat oven to 200°F. Remove the tofu from it's packaging and wrap it with paper towels. Place a plate on top to weigh it down. I used a large tin of vegetables in this picture, but you can use anything handy. Let the tofu sit for a while to press some of the water out.

Place about 1/4 cup of cilantro, 3 tbsp rice vinegar, 2 tbsp toasted sesame oil, minced garlic, crushed red pepper flakes, and transfer to a large mixing bowl. Whisk everything together.

Peel and julienne the eggplant. You can julienne roughly by hand like I did, or you can use a mandolin with a julienne attachment for more precise "noodles." Place the eggplant into the marinade.

Add olive oil to a skillet over medium-low heat and cook the eggplant until it softens. Keep in mind that the eggplant absorbs liquid, so if you have issues with it sticking to the pan, feel free to add a little bit more sesame or olive oil - just be sure to adjust your nutrition tracking.

Turn the oven off. Combine the remaining cilantro with the eggplant and transfer the noodles to an oven safe dish. Cover with a lid or foil, and place into the oven to keep warm. Clean out the skillet and return to the stovetop to heat up again.

Unwrap the tofu and cut it into 8 even slices. Spread the sesame seeds on a plate. Press both sides of each piece of tofu into the seeds to act as a crust.

Add 2 tbsps of sesame oil to the skillet. Fry both sides of the tofu for 5 minutes each, or until they start to crisp up. Pour the 1/4 cup of soy sauce into the pan and coat the pieces of tofu. Cook until the tofu slices look browned and caramelized with the soy sauce.

Remove the noodles from the oven and top with tofu.

ZUCCHINI RIBBONS & AVOCADO WALNUT PESTO

Ingredients
Zucchini Ribbons
3 medium zucchini
1/2 tsp salt

Avocado Walnut Pesto
1/2 large avocado
1 cup fresh basil leaves
1/4 cup walnuts
2 cloves garlic, peeled
1/2 large lemon
1/4 cup grated Parmesan cheese
1/2 cup water, if needed*

Other
1 tbsp olive oil
5-6 fresh basil leaves to garnish
Salt and pepper to taste

Directions
Cut the zucchini into delicate ribbons with a vegetable peeler or mandolin slicer, being careful to stop peeling once you reach the seeds.
Place the ribbons in a colander and toss with salt. Let stand while you prepare the avocado pesto.
Gather the avocado walnut pesto ingredients.

Add all ingredients into a food processor and blend until the sauce is smooth. If your sauce is too thick, you can add water to thin it as needed.

Grease a skillet with 1 tbsp olive oil and bring to medium heat.

Saute zucchini ribbons for 3-5 minutes or until they just begin to soften. Remove from heat.

Spoon pesto onto zucchini ribbons and gently toss to coat.

Plate two portions of fantastically swirled vegetable ribbons and garnish with fresh basil and grated Parmesan cheese.

LOW CARB FRIED MAC & CHEESE

Ingredients
1 medium cauliflower, riced
1 1/2 cups shredded cheddar cheese
3 large eggs
2 tsps paprika
1 tsp turmeric
3/4 tsp rosemary

Directions
Rice the cauliflower in a food processor then cook it in the microwave for 5 minutes.
Dry it out by wringing it in a kitchen towel or paper towels; you want as little moisture as possible.
Add your eggs one by one followed by cheese and spices to the cauliflower and mix together.
Heat olive oil and coconut oil in a pan on high heat.
Form small patties out of the cauliflower mixture.
Fry on both sides until crisp.

TOMATO BASIL AND MOZZARELLA GALETTE

Ingredients
1 cup almond flour
1 large egg
3 tbsp mozzarella liquid
1 tsp garlic powder
1/4 cup shredded Parmesan cheese
2 tbsp pesto
3-4 fresh basil leaves
1/2 ounce Mozzarella pearls*
3-4 cherry tomatoes

Directions
Heat oven to 375°F and line a cookie sheet with parchment, spraying it with non stick spray. Combine the almond flour, garlic powder, and mozzarella liquid in a bowl, stirring gently.
Add the egg and Parmesan cheese, then mix well until dough forms.
Form the dough mixture into a large ball and place on the prepared parchment.
Press the dough ball into a circle, working to keep the thickness uniform. It should press out to about 1/2 inch thick. It may be sticky, so wetting your hands with water can help keep your fingers from sticking to the crust.
Spread pesto evenly over the center of the crust, leaving room to fold in the edges. Layer mozzarella, basil leaves, and tomatoes.

Using the edge of the parchment, fold the edges of the crust up and over the filling. Work in a circle around the edge until all of the edges are folded up.

Bake for 20 to 25 minutes or until the crust is golden brown and the cheese is melted.

KETO GRILLED CHEESE SANDWICH

Ingredients
Bun *Ingredient*s
2 large eggs
2 tbsp almond flour
1 1/2 tbsps psyllium husk powder
1/2 tsp baking powder
2 tbsp butter, softened

Fillings & Extras
2 ounces cheddar cheese
1 tbsp butter

Directions
Mix all of the bun ingredients together in a bowl and mix until it thickens up.
Pour mixture into a square bowl or container and level it off. Clean sides if needed.
Microwave for 90 seconds. If more time is needed, continue cooking in 15 second intervals.
Once cooked, remove bread from container and slice in half.
Put cheese between bun, heat butter in a pan over medium heat, and fry the grilled cheese until you are happy with the texture.

FRESH BELL PEPPER BASIL PIZZA

Ingredients
Pizza Base
6 ounces mozzarella cheese
1/2 cup almond flour
2 tbsp psyllium husk
2 tbsps cream cheese
2 tbsps fresh Parmesan cheese
1 large egg
1 tsp Italian seasoning
1/2 tsp salt
1/2 tsp pepper

Toppings
4 ounces shredded cheddar cheese
1 medium vine tomato
1/4 cup Rao's Marinara Sauce
2/3 medium bell pepper
2-3 tbsp fresh chopped basil

Directions
1. Preheat oven to 400F.
2. Microwave mozarella cheese for 40-50 seconds or until completely melted and pliable.
3. Add the rest of the pizza ingredients (EXCEPT for toppings) to the cheese and mix together well. I recommend using your hands.
4. Using your hands or a rolling pin, flatten the dough and form a circle.

5. Bake for 10 minutes and remove pizza from the oven. Top the pizza with the toppings and bake for another 8-10 minutes.
6. Remove pizza from the oven and let cool.

KETO BREAKFAST BROWNIE MUFFINS

Ingredients

1 cup golden flaxseed meal
1/4 cup cocoa powder
1 tbsp cinnamon
1/2 tbsp baking powder
1/2 tsp salt
1 large egg
2 tbsp coconut oil
1/4 cup sugar-free caramel syrup
1/2 cup pumpkin puree
1 tsp vanilla extract
1 tsp apple cider vinegar
1/4 cup slivered almonds

Directions

Preheat your oven to 350°F and combine all ingredients in a deep mixing bowl and mix to combine.

Line a muffin tin with 6 paper liners and spoon about 1/4 cup of batter into each muffin liner.

Sprinkle slivered almonds over the top of each muffin and press gently so that they stay.

Bake in the oven for about 15 minutes. You should see the muffins rise and set on top.

VEGETARIAN GREEK COLLARD WRAPS

Ingredients
Tzatziki Sauce
1 cup plain Greek yogurt, full-fat
1 tsp garlic powder
1 tbsp white vinegar
2 tbsp olive oil
2.5 ounces (1/4) cucumber, seeded and grated
2 tbsp minced fresh dill
Salt and pepper to taste

The Wrap
4 large collard green leaves, washed
1 medium cucumber, julienned
1/2 medium red bell pepper, julienned
1/2 cup purple onion, diced
8 kalamata olives, halved
1/2 block (4-oz) feta, cut into 4 (1-inch thick) strips
4 cherry tomatoes, halved

Directionss
Mix all of the ingredients for the tzatziki sauce together then store it in the fridge. Be sure to squeeze all of the water out of the cucumber after you grate it.
Prepare collard green wraps by washing leaves well and trimming the fibrous stem from each leaf.
Spread 2 tbsp of tzatziki onto the center of each wrap and smooth the sauce out.

Layer the cucumber, pepper, onion, olives, feta, and tomatoes in the center of the wrap. I've shown them spread out in a line to display each ingredient, but when assembling these wraps, it works best to keep all of the ingredients close and toward the center of the leaf. Imagine piling them high rather than spreading them out!

Fold as you would a burrito, folding in each side toward the center and the folding the rounded end over the filling and roll.

You can slice the wraps in half and serve with any leftover tzatziki or save it as a leftover meal!

SUN DRIED TOMATO PESTO MUG CAKE

Ingredients
Base
1 large egg
2 tbsps butter
2 tbsp almond flour
1/2 tsp baking powder

Flavor
5 tsps sun dried tomato pesto
1 tbsp almond flour
Pinch salt

Directions
Mix all ingredients together.
Microwave for 75 seconds on high (power level 10).
You can either lightly tap the cup against plate to take the mug cake out or you can take a butter knife around the edges of the cake to loosen it. Add extra tomato pesto and serve!

SESAME ALMOND ZOODLE BOWL

Ingredients
Zoodles
2 medium zucchini, spiralized
1/2 cup sliced mushrooms
1 cup shredded broccoli slaw*
1 tsp sesame oil

Sauce
1/4 cup almond butter
2 tbsp soy sauce
2 tbsp sesame oil
1/4 tsp garlic powder
1 tsp crushed red pepper flakes
1 tsp erythritol
2 tbsp chopped almonds, garnish
Optional: Pinch of chili powder

Directions
Heat 1 tsp of sesame oil in a large skillet on medium heat. Add the shredded broccoli and cabbage mix along with the mushrooms and sauté until they begin to soften.

Make your zucchini noodles using a vegetable spiralizer and pat them dry with a towel to remove some of the excess moisture.

Add your zoodles to the skillet and heat evenly by gently turning the zoodles with a fork or tongs until the noodles become soft but not soggy, about 3-5 minutes.

Make your sauce by adding all ingredients in a large bowl and combining thoroughly.

Add a touch more water or oil if necessary to reach your desired consistency.

Portion your zoodles in three bowls and drizzle with sesame almond sauce then toss to coat.

Top with chopped almonds and crushed red pepper flakes and an optional pinch of chili powder.

CHEESY THYME WAFFLES

Ingredients
1/2 large head cauliflower, riced
1 cup finely shredded mozzarella cheese
1 cup packed collard greens
1/3 cup Parmesan cheese
2 large eggs
2 stalks green onion
1 tbsp sesame seed
1 tbsp olive oil
2 tsps fresh chopped thyme
1 tsp garlic powder
1/2 tsp ground black pepper
1/2 tsp salt

Directions
Rice the cauliflower by pulsing the florets in a food processor until a crumbly texture is achieved.
Add collard greens, spring onion, and thyme, then continue pulsing until everything is well combined.
Scoop the mixture out into a mixing bowl, add the rest of the ingredients, and mix together well.
Spoon mixture evenly over the griddle of a waffle iron once it's hot.
Cook the waffle according to your waffle makers' manufacturing instructions, then remove.

CHEESY HEARTS OF PALM DIP

Ingredients
1 (14-ounce) can hearts of palm, drained
3 green onions stalks, chopped
1/4 cup mayonnaise
2 tbsp Italian seasoning
1/2 cup Parmesan cheese, shredded
2 large eggs, separate 1 of the eggs

Topping
1/4 cup Parmesan cheese

Directions
Heat oven to 350°F and prepare a small baking dish with nonstick spray.
Chop the green onion bulbs and drain your hearts of palm. It is not necessary to cut the palm before adding it to your food processor, but it can help if you have an older or less powerful model.
Combine the Hearts of Palm, onion, seasoning, Parmesan cheese, and mayo in the food processor. Pulse until the mixture is smooth.
Add one whole egg and one egg yolk to the processor. Pulse three to four times to combine.
Pour the dip into prepared baking dish and cook for 15 – 20 minutes or until the mixture begins to puff up slightly. Stir and top with more Parmesan cheese.
Broil until the cheese is melted and begins to brown. Serve hot with veggies or keto crackers.

LOW CARB BROCCOLI AND CHEESE FRITTERS

Ingredients
Fritters
3/4 cup almond flour
1/4 cup + 3 tbsp flaxseed meal
4 ounces fresh broccoli
4 ounces mozzarella cheese
2 large eggs
2 tsps baking powder
Salt and Pepper to taste

Sauce
1/4 cup mayonnaise
1/4 cup fresh chopped dill
1/2 tbsp lemon juice
Salt and pepper to taste

Directions
Add broccoli to a food processor and process until broccoli is completely broken down.
Add cheese, almond flour, 1/4 cup flaxseed meal, and baking powder. If you want to add any extra seasonings (salt and pepper), so at this point.
Add the eggs and mix together well until everything is incorperated.
Roll the batter into balls and then coat with 3 tbsp flaxseed meal.
Heat your deep fryer to 375F and lay fritters inside the basket, not overcrowing it.

Fry the fritters until they are golden brown, about 3-5 minutes. Once done, lay them on paper towels to drain excess grease and season to your tastes.

If desired, you can make a zesty dill and lemon mayonnaise for a dip. Enjoy!

WARM ASIAN BROCCOLI SALAD

Ingredients

12 ounce bag broccoli slaw
2 tbsps coconut oil
1 tbsp coconut aminos
1 tsp fresh ginger, grated
1/2 tsp salt
1/4 tsp pepper
1/2 cup full fat plain goat milk yogurt
1/2 tbsp sesame seeds
Cilantro, as an optional garnish

Direction

Preheat coconut oil in a large skillet over medium high heat. Place the broccoli slaw into the skillet, cover, and cook for 7 minutes.

Remove the lid fro the skillet and stir in the coconut aminos, ginger, salt and pepper. Remove your skillet from the heat, then stir in yogurt and top with sesame seeds. Garnish with cilantro, if desired.

CAULIFLOWER MAC & CHEESE

Ingredients
2 pounds frozen cauliflower florets
1 cup heavy whipping cream
4 ounces cream cheese, cubed
8 ounces cheddar cheese, shredded
1 tsps Dijon mustard
1 tsp turmeric
1/2 tsp powdered garlic
Salt and pepper to taste

Directions
Cook the cauliflower florets according to the package instructions.
Bring the cream to a simmer. Then, use a whisk to stir in the cream cheese and mix until smooth.
Stir in 6 ounces of the shredded cheddar cheese, saving the other 2 ounces for later. Mix until the cheese melts into the sauce.
Add the Dijon mustard, turmeric, powdered garlic, salt, and pepper. The sauce will become a smooth yellow color.
Make sure that the cauliflower is drained, then add it to the cheese sauce. Evenly coat the florets with sauce.
Sprinkle on the remaining 2 ounces of cheddar cheese, then stir until mostly melted.

PERSONAL PAN PIZZA DIP

Ingredients
Personal Pan Pizza Dip
4 ounces cream cheese
1/4 cup sour cream
1/4 cup mayonnaise
1 cup shredded mozzarella cheese
Salt and pepper to taste
1/2 cup Rao's tomato sauce
1/4 cup Parmesan cheese

Pepperoni, Peppers, and Olives
6 slices pepperoni, chopped
1 tbsp diced green pepper
4 pitted sliced black olives
1/2 tsp Italian seasoning
Salt and pepper to taste

Mushrooms and Peppers
1 tbsp diced green pepper
2 tbsp diced baby bella mushrooms
1/2 tsp Italian seasoning
Salt and pepper to taste

Directions
Pre-heat oven to 350F. Measure out the cream cheese and microwave for 20 seconds or leave it out until it is room temperature.

Mix the sour cream, mayonnaise, and mozzarella cheese into the cream cheese. Season with salt and pepper to taste.

Divide the mixture between 4 ramekins, then spoon 2 tbsp of tomato sauce over each ramekin.

Measure out 1/2 cup mozzarella cheese and 1/4 cup parmesan cheese, then sprinkle mixture over the the sauce evenly.

Add toppings of choice to your personal pan pizza dips.

Bake for 18-20 minutes or until cheese is bubbling.

Remove from oven and let cool.

VEGETARIAN THREE CHEESE QUICHE STUFFED PEPPERS

Ingredients
2 medium bell peppers, halved and seeded
4 large eggs
1/2 cup ricotta cheese
1/2 cup shredded mozzarella
1/2 cup grated Parmesan cheese
1 tsp garlic powder
1/4 tsp dried parsley
1/4 cup baby spinach leaves
2 tbsp Parmesan cheese, to garnish

Directions
Heat oven to 375°F. Prepare the peppers by slicing them into four equal halves and removing the seeds.

In a small food processor, blend the three cheeses, eggs, garlic powder, and parsley. My food processor is smaller than I would like, so I did this in two batches, half and half, and then combined both fillings.

Pour the egg mixture into each pepper, filling just below the rim. Place a few baby spinach leaves on top and stir with a fork, pushing them under the egg.

Cover with foil and bake for 35-45 minutes or until the egg is set.

Sprinkle with Parmesan cheese and broil for 3-5 minutes or until the tops begin to brown.

ROASTED MUSHROOM AND WALNUT CAULIFLOWER GRITS

Ingredients

6 ounces baby portobello mushrooms, sliced
3 cloves garlic, minced
1 tbsp rosemary
1/2 cup chopped walnuts
1 tbsp smoked paprika
2 tbsp olive oil
1 medium head of cauliflower
1/2 cup water
1 cup half-and-half
1 cup shredded sharp cheddar
2 tbsp butter
Salt to taste

Directions

Heat oven to 400°F and line a cookie sheet with foil. Combine the sliced mushrooms, minced garlic, rosemary, walnuts, and smoked paprika in a small dish and drizzle with olive oil. Toss to coat and season with salt.

Spread the mixture evenly on the cookie sheet and roast in the oven for 15 minutes.

Process one head of cauliflower florets in a food processor by pulsing it until it is very fine.

Steam the processed cauliflower in a medium pot, covered, with 1/2 cup water for 5 minutes or until the mixture is slightly tender. You don't want it to be too soft since it will need to resemble grits.

Pour half-and-half into the cauliflower grits, stir, and simmer on medium-low heat for 3 minutes or just until the milk is heated.

Stir in the sharp cheddar and butter and reduce heat to low until the mixture is creamy and well combined. Season with salt to taste. If you like your grits runny add another 1/4 cup of water.

Remove roasting pan from the oven once the mushrooms are soft and the edges are a deep brown.

Serve the cauliflower grits hot, and top with the mushroom mixture and extra butter if desired.

CHARRED VEGGIE AND FRIED GOAT CHEESE SALAD

Ingredients
   2 tbsp poppy seeds
   2 tbsp sesame seeds
   1 tsp onion flakes
   1 tsp garlic flakes
   4 ounces goat cheese, cut into 4 1/2 in thick medallions
   1 medium red bell pepper, seeds removed & cut into 8 pieces
   1/2 cup baby portobello mushrooms, sliced
   4 cups arugula, divided between two bowls
   1 tbsp avocado oil

Directions
1. Combine the poppy and sesame seeds, onion, and garlic flakes in a small dish.
2. Coat each piece of goat cheese on both sides then plate and place in the refrigerator until you are ready to fry the cheese.
3. Prepare a skillet with nonstick spray and bring to medium heat. Char the peppers and mushrooms on both sides, just until the pieces begin to darken and the pepper softens. Add to the bowls of arugula.
4. Place the cold goat cheese in the skillet and fry on each side for about 30 seconds. This melts quickly so be gentle as you flip each piece!
5. Add the cheese to the salad and drizzle with avocado oil. Serve warm!

CRISPY TOFU AND BOK CHOY SALAD

Ingredients
- 15 ounces extra firm tofu
- 1 tbsp soy sauce
- 1 tbsp sesame oil
- 1 tbsp water
- 2 tsps minced garlic
- 1 tbsp rice wine vinegar
- Juice of 1/2 lemon

Bok Choy Salad
- 9 ounces bok choy
- 1 stalk green onion
- 2 tbsp chopped cilantro
- 3 tbsp coconut oil
- 2 tbsp soy sauce
- 1 tbsp sambal olek
- 1 tbsp peanut butter
- Juice 1/2 lime
- 7 drops liquid stevia

Directions
1. Start by pressing the tofu by placing it in a kitchen towel with something heavy over the top (like a cast iron skillet). This is a long process as it takes about 4-6 hours to dry out. Additionally, you may need to replace the kitchen towel half-way through.

2. Once the tofu is pressed, start your marinade by combining all of the ingredients for the marinade (soy sauce, sesame oil, water, garlic, vinegar, and lemon).

3. Chop the tofu into squares and place in a plastic bag along with the marinade. Let this marinate for at least 30 minutes, but preferably over night.

4. Pre-heat oven to 350°F. Place tofu on a baking sheet lined with parchment paper (or a silpat) and bake for 30-35 minutes.

5. As the tofu cooks, get started on the bok choy salad by chopping cilantro and spring onion.

6. Mix all of the other ingredients together (except lime juice and bok choy) in a bowl. Then add cilantro and spring onion.

Note: You can microwave coconut oil for 10-15 seconds to allow it it to melt.

7. Once the tofu is almost cooked, add lime juice into the salad dressing and mix together.

8. Chop the bok choy into small slices, like you would cabbage.

9. Remove the tofu from the oven and assemble your salad with tofu, bok choy, and sauce.

VEGETARIAN GREEK COLLARD WRAPS

Ingredients

Tzatziki Sauce
1 cup plain Greek yogurt, full-fat
1 tsp garlic powder
1 tbsp white vinegar
2 tbsp olive oil
2.5 ounces (1/4) cucumber, seeded and grated
2 tbsps minced fresh dill
Salt and pepper to taste

The Wrap
4 large collard green leaves, washed
1 medium cucumber, julienned
1/2 medium red bell pepper, julienned
1/2 cup purple onion, diced
8 kalamata olives, halved
1/2 block (4-oz) feta, cut into 4 (1-inch thick) strips
4 cherry tomatoes, halved

Directions

Mix all of the ingredients for the tzatziki sauce together and store it in the fridge.

Note: Be sure to squeeze all of the water out of the cucumber after you grate it.

Prepare collard green wraps by washing the leaves well and trimming the fibrous stem from each leaf.

Spread 2 tbsps of tzatziki onto the center of each wrap and smooth the sauce out.

Layer the cucumber, peppers, onion, olives, feta, and tomatoes in the center of the wrap. I've shown them spread out in a line to display each ingredient, but when assembling these wraps, it actually works best to keep all of the ingredients close and toward the center of the leaf. Imagine piling them high rather than spreading them out!

Fold the wrap the same way that you fold a burrito, brinigng in each side toward the center and the folding the rounded end over the filling and roll.

Slice in half and serve with any leftover tzatziki or wrap in plastic for easy leftovers.

Notes

Nutrition breakdown accounts for approximately 2 tbsp of tzatziki per wrap.

SESAME ALMOND ZOODLE BOWL

Ingredients
Zoodles
- 2 medium zucchini, spiralized
- 1/2 cup sliced mushrooms
- 1 cup shredded broccoli slaw
- 1 tsp sesame oil

Sauce
- 1/4 cup almond butter
- 2 tbsp soy sauce
- 2 tbsp sesame oil
- 1/4 tsp garlic powder
- 1 tsp crushed red pepper flakes
- 1 tsp erythritol
- 2 tbsp chopped almonds, garnish

Optional: pinch of chili powder

Directions
1. Heat 1 tsp of sesame oil in a large skillet on medium heat. Add the shredded broccoli cabbage mix and mushrooms, then sauté until they begin to soften.
2. Make your zucchini noodles using a vegetable spiralizer and pat them dry with a towel to remove excess moisture.
3. Add your zoodles to the skillet and heat evenly by gently turning the zoodles with a fork or tongs until the noodles become soft but not soggy, about 3-5 minutes.

4. Mix your sauce by adding all ingredients in a large bowl and combining thoroughly.

5. If you desire a thinner consistency, you ca nadd more water or oil.

6. Portion your zoodles in three bowls and drizzle with sesame almond sauce then toss to coat.

7. Top with chopped almonds and crushed red pepper flakes and an optional pinch of chili powder.

VEGETARIAN THREE CHEESE QUICHE STUFFED PEPPERS

Ingredients
- 2 medium bell peppers, sliced in half and seeded
- 4 large eggs
- 1/2 cup ricotta cheese
- 1/2 cup shredded mozzarella
- 1/2 cup grated Parmesan cheese
- 1 tsp garlic powder
- 1/4 tsp dried parsley
- 1/4 cup baby spinach leaves
- 2 tbsps Parmesan cheese, to garnish

Directions

1. Heat oven to 375°F. Prepare the peppers by slicing them each into equal halves. Remove the seeds.
2. In a small food processor, blend the three cheeses, eggs, garlic powder, and parsley. My food processor is smaller than I would like so I did this in two batches, half and half, and then combined both fillings.
3. Pour the egg mixture into each pepper, filling just below the rim. Place baby spinach leaves on top and stir with a fork, pushing them under the egg. Cover with foil and bake for 35-45 minutes or until the egg is set.
4. Sprinkle with Parmesan cheese and broil for 3-5 minutes or until the tops begin to brown

VEGETARIAN RED COCONUT CURRY

Ingredients
1 cup broccoli florets
1 large handful of spinach
4 tbsp coconut oil
1/4 medium onion
1 tsp minced garlic
1 tsp minced ginger
2 tsps Fish sauce
2 tsps soy sauce
1 tbsp red curry paste
1/2 cup coconut cream (or coconut milk)

Directions
Chop onions and minced garlic. Add 2 tbsp of coconut oil to a pan and bring it to medium-high heat.

Once hot, add the onions to the pan and cook until they are semi-translucent. Then, add garlic to the the pan until fragrant.

Turn heat down to medium-low and add broccoli to the pan, stirring everything well together.

Once broccoli is partially cooked, move vegetables to the side of the pan and add curry paste. Let this cook for 45-60 seconds.

Add spinach and once it begins to wilt, add the coconut cream along with the rest of the coconut oil.

Stir together and add soy sauce, fish sauce, and ginger. Let simmer for 5-10 minutes or until the sauce reaches your desired consistency.

VEGAN KETO PORRIDGE

Ingredients

    2 tbsp coconut flour
    3 tbsp golden flaxseed meal
    2 tbsps vegan vanilla protein powder*
    1 1/2 cups unsweetened almond milk
    Powdered erythritol to taste

Note: Try experimenting with different flavors!

Directions

1. In a bowl, mix together the coconut flour, golden flaxseed meal, and protein powder.
2. Add to a sauce pan along with the almond milk and cook over medium heat.
3. It will seem very loose at first, but when it thickens, you can stir in your preferred amount of sweetener. I like to use about 1/2 a tbsp. Serve with your favorite toppings.

LEMON RASPBERRY SWEET ROLLS

Ingredients
Lemon cream cheese filling
4 oz cream cheese, room temperature
2 tbsp butter, room temperature
2 tbsp stevia erythritol blend*
1/2 tsp vanilla extract
1 tsp lemon extract
Zest from one lemon (about 2 tsps)
1 tsp Lemon juice

Raspberry sauce:
2 tbsp stevia erythritol blend*
1/4 tsp xanthan gum
1 tbsp water
2 tsps lemon juice
1/2 cup frozen raspberries

Dough:
1 cup super fine almond flour
1/4 cup stevia erythritol blend*
1/4 tsp zanthan gum
1 1/4 tsp baking powder
1 large egg
1 tsp vanilla extract
2 cups part-skim mozzarella cheese

Lemon glaze (optional)
2 tbsp butter, room temperature

1/2 ounce cream cheese, room temperature
1/4 tsp vanilla extract
2 tbsp stevia erythritol blend*
1 tsp lemon juice
1/4 tsp lemon extract
1 1/2 tbsp unsweetened almond milk, room temperature

Directions
Lemon Cream Cheese Filling:
Use an electric mixer to beat the cream cheese, butter, sweetener, vanilla extract, lemon extract, lemon zest, and lemon juice until smooth. Set aside.
Raspberry Sauce:
In a medium saucepan, whisk together sweetener and xanthan gum. Gradually add water and lemon juice while whisking.
Set heat to medium-low and add frozen raspberries, stirring constantly. Just when the sauce begins to simmer, remove from heat and set aside.
Dough:
Preheat oven to 350F degrees. Spray a 9" circular pan with coconut oil or grease with butter. Have two 15 inch sheets of parchment and a rolling pin handy.
Prepare a double boiler – a medium saucepan with a medium bowl that will sit on top works fine for this purpose. Add about 2 inches of water to the saucepan or the bottom part of the double boiler. Place over high heat and bring to a simmer uncovered. Once it begins to simmer, reduce heat to low.

Meanwhile in the top-part of the double boiler (with it not over the water), combine the almond flour, stevia/erythritol sweetener, xanthan gum, and baking powder using a whisk.

Stir in the egg and vanilla extract. Keep in mind that the mixture will be very thick.

Stir in the mozzarella cheese and place the bowl over the pot of simmering water. Be sure to protect your hands from the hot bowl and the steam escaping the pot (a silicone mitten works well for this purpose).

Stir the mixture constantly while the cheese melts and combines with the flour. It will begin to look like bread dough.

When the cheese has melted completely, transfer the dough to a prepared piece of parchment paper. Knead the dough until the flour is completely combined with with the cheese. Pat dough into a rectangular shape and cover with the second piece of parchment. Roll out dough into about 12" X 15" rectangle.

Remove top parchment.

Evenly spread the lemon cream cheese filling on the dough, leaving about 1/2 inch uncovered on the edges, then spread the raspberry sauce over the lemon cream cheese filling.

Starting at the long side, roll the dough into a log shape.Press the outside long edge to seal.

Using a serrated knife, gently cut the log crosswise into 8 pieces. Arrange rolls in the prepared pan with one roll in the center and the rest circled around it.

Bake for 24-26 minutes, or until golden brown.

Lemon glaze:

In a small bowl, beat butter and cream cheese with an electric mixer until smooth.

Add vanilla, sweetener, lemon juice, and lemon extract until incorporated.

Gradually add the almond milk, one tsp at a time, beating the mixture between each addition.

KETO BREAKFAST BROWNIE MUFFINS

Ingredients
- 1 cup golden flaxseed meal
- 1/4 cup cocoa powder
- 1 tbsp cinnamon
- 1/2 tbsp baking powder
- 1/2 tsp salt
- 1 large egg
- 2 tbsp coconut oil
- 1/4 cup sugar-free caramel syrup
- 1/2 cup pumpkin puree
- 1 tsp vanilla extract
- 1 tsp apple cider vinegar
- 1/4 cup slivered almonds

Directions

1. Preheat your oven to 350°F and combine all your dry *ingredients* in a deep mixing bowl; mix to combine.
2. In a separate bowl, combine all your wet ingredients.
3. Combine you wet ingredients with your dry ingredients and mix well.
4. Line a muffin tin with paper liners and spoon about 1/4 cup of batter into each muffin liner. This recipe should yield 6 muffins. Sprinkle slivered almonds over the top of each muffin and press gently so that they stick.
5. Bake in the oven for about 15 minutes. You should see the muffins rise and set on top. Enjoy warm or cool.

AVOCADO CHOCOLATE MOUSSE

Ingredients

4 ounces chopped semisweet chocolate or chocolate chips (at least 60% dark), about 1/2 cup plus 2 tbsps

2 large, ripe avocados

3 tbsps unsweetened cocoa powder

1/4 cup Almond Breeze Unsweetened Almondmilk Cashewmilk Blend

1 tsp pure vanilla extract

1/8 tsp kosher salt

For serving: fresh raspberries, sliced strawberries, whipped cream (or whipped coconut cream to keep vegan), and chocolate shavings

Directions

Place the chopped chocolate or chocolate chips in a microwave-safe bowl. Microwave in 15-second increments, stirring between each and watching carefully so that the chocolate does not burn. When the chocolate is almost completely melted, remove it from the microwave and stir until smooth. Set aside and let cool until just barely warm.

Halve and pit the avocados, then scoop them into a food processor fitted with a steel blade. Add the melted chocolate, cocoa powder, almond milk/cashew milk blend, vanilla extract, and salt. Blend until very smooth and creamy, stopping to scrape down the bowl as needed. Taste and add a few teaspoons of agave if you would like it to be a bit sweeter. Spoon into glasses. Enjoy immediately as a pudding, or for a thicker, mousse-like consistency, refrigerate until well chilled, 2 hours or overnight. Serve topped with raspberries, cream, and chocolate shavings.

CAULIFLOWER SOUP

Ingredients

   3 tsps olive oil
   1 1/2 pounds cauliflower, roughly chopped
   1 1/4 cups green cabbage, roughly chopped
   1/2 cup leeks, roughly chopped
   2 tbsp garlic, minced
   1/2 cup parsnip, roughly chopped
   1 1/2 tsps rosemary, minced
   3/4 tsp thyme leaves
   2 cups coconut milk
   2 1/2 cups celery juice (or vegetable stock)
   1 tsp Himalayan salt (additional to taste)
   Black pepper, freshly cracked, to taste
   Nutmeg, to taste

Directions

Heat the oil in the stock pot, and sauté the cauliflower, leeks, parsnips, garlic, rosemary, and thyme until the cauliflower is slightly browned.

Add the celery juice (or vegetable stock) and coconut milk and let it simmer for approximately 30 minutes. Season with salt, pepper, and nutmeg.

Blend until smooth, either using a handheld immersion blender or transferring your soup to a food processor or blender in 2 or 3 batches (depending on the size of the blender.)

CHEESY EGG MUFFINS

Ingredients
  1 dozen eggs
  1/2 tsp sea salt
  Ghee or nonstick cooking spray, to coat pans
  1 cup frozen or fresh spinach
  1 heaping cup thinly sliced mushrooms
  1/4 cup thinly sliced green onion
  1 1/2 to 2 cups shredded cheese (either cheddar or parmesan)

Directions
Preheat the oven to 350°F. Crack eggs into a liquid measuring cup and whisk them with salt.
Grease a 12-cup muffin pan with butter or ghee. Divide spinach, mushrooms, green onion, and cheese between each muffin cup, then carefully pour eggs over tops until muffin tins are almost full (leave 1/4-inch of space).
Bake for 20-25 minutes or until a wooden pick, knife, etc. that is inserted in the center of a muffin comes out clean. The egg muffins will look like soufflé when they come out of the oven, but will sink after a few minutes. Let them rest in the muffin tin for a few minutes before carefully removing each muffin using a rubber spatula.
Serve immediately or let cool and transfer to a resealable plastic bag. Refrigerate for up to a week or freeze for a month.

ITALIAN BAKED EGG AND VEGETABLES

Ingredients

   1 pound plum tomatoes, cut into 1-inch chunks
   1 red bell pepper, cut into 3/4-inch pieces
   1 zucchini, quartered lengthwise, cut crosswise into 3/4-inch chunks
   1 onion, halved lengthwise, sliced
   2 large garlic cloves, minced
   1/2 tsp dried basil (or 1/2 tbsp fresh)
   1/2 tsp salt
   1/4 tsp black pepper
   4 large eggs
   1/4 cup grated fat-free parmesan cheese

Directions

Heat oven to 400°F, and cover a shallow roasting pan with nonstick cooking spray. Put the tomatoes, bell pepper, zucchini, onion, garlic, basil, salt, and pepper in pan and also spray with nonstick spray (or use olive oil). Toss to coat. Roast, stirring occasionally, until vegetables are browned and tender, about 30 minutes.

Spray four 8 or 10 ounce ramekins or custard cups with nonstick spray. Divide roasted vegetables evenly among cups. Make a well in the center of the vegetables, and carefully break one egg into each cup. Sprinkle with parmesan cheese. Place cups on baking sheet, and bake until eggs are just set, about 20 to 25 minutes.

KETO TABBOULEH

Ingredients
- 1/2 cup (120 ml) extra-virgin olive oil
- 1/4 cup (80 ml) lemon juice
- 1/2 tsp gray sea salt
- 2 bunches of fresh parsley, chopped
- 1⅓ cup (215 g) Manitoba Harvest Hemp Hearts
- 3 medium tomatoes, diced
- 8 green onions, finely diced
- 1/4 cup (24 g) chopped fresh mint
- 1 small garlic clove, minced

Directions
Place the olive oil, lemon juice and sea salt in a large bowl, Whisk to combine.
Add remaining ingredients and toss to coat. Serve

VEGAN KETO COOKIE CARAMEL COOKIE BARS

Ingredients
  1/2 cup (112g) coconut oil, softened
  1/2 cup unsweetened coconut milk or preferred non-dairy milk
  2 tbsp (10g) whole psyllium husk
  2 tbsp (24g) golden granulated sweetener
  1/4 tsp salt
  1 tsp vanilla extract
  1/2 cup (50g) coconut flour
  1/2 cup (30g) unsweetened coconut flakes
  1/2 cup (56g) raw macadamia nut halves
  1 ounce (30g) unsweetened baking chocolate
  1/4 cup (60ml) Coconut Dulce de Leche

Directions
Preheat the oven to 350°F (177°C) and line an 8"x8" (20cm x 20cm) brownie pan with parchment paper, leaving at least 2" (5cm) extra on two opposing sides to make it easier to remove them form the pan.

In a medium mixing bowl, mix the coconut oil, coconut milk, psyllium, granulated sweetener, salt and vanilla until completely combined and smooth. This takes about a minute of stirring.

Next, add the coconut flour, coconut flakes, macadamia nuts and chocolate and stir until everything is evenly distributed. The dough will resemble a drop cookie dough batter.

Press the dough evenly into the brownie pan and bake for 30 minutes or until the peaks begin to turn golden and the dough is firm to the touch.

Remove from the pan using the extra parchment as handles and let cool for an hour so the bars have time to set up. You can also speed this process up by putting the bars in the freezer for about 15 minutes .

Once cooled, slice into 9 equal portions and either drizzle or pipe the Quick Coconut Dulce de Leche on top.

To store the bars, refrigerate them in a covered container for up to four days or freeze for up to a month.

KETO COCONUT DULCE DE LECHE

Ingredients
   2 cans (13.5oz/400ml each) coconut milk, full fat
   1/4 cup, plus 1 tbsp (60g) granulated sweetener
   1/4 tsp saltu8

Directions
In a large saucepan on medium-high heat, stir ingredients together. Heat for about five minutes, whisking occasionally until the mixture begins to boil.

Turn the heat down to medium and continue whisking frequently making sure that you whisk away the "foam" that appears. Once this foam is completely gone (about 13-14 minutes), cook for another minute, whisking constantly. This will bring the cooking time to about 20 minutes total.

The dulce de leche will have thickened to a caramel consistency and will be a medium golden color.

Let it cool for about ten minutes before either using or transferring to a heat-safe jar and continuing to cool, uncovered, in the fridge. Once cool, cover and store.

To store, refrigerate in a sealed jar for up to two weeks.

To reheat, scoop the caramel into a small saucepan on low heat and gently heat for about five minutes, whisking occasionally, until the caramel becomes smooth and pourable.

VEGAN KETO MAPLE CINNAMON NOATMEAL

Ingredients
  3 tbsp (30g) hulled hemp seeds
  3 tbsp (30g) Vega Clean Protein in vanilla
  2 tbsp (15g) ground flax seeds
  1/2 tsp ground cinnamon
  2 tbsp Lakanto sugar-free maple syrup
  3/4 cup (180ml) hot water

Directions
Stir dry ingredients together in a bowl. Next, pour the water over, and continue stirring until the lumps are gone. The mixture will continue to thicken as it cools.
Top with sugar-free maple syrup.

PANCAKE MUFFINS

Ingredients:
    1/2 cup plain yogurt, whole milk
    2 tbsp coconut oil or unsalted butter, melted
    1 tsp vanilla extract
    1/4 tsp apple cider vinegar
    1 3/4 cup almond flour
    1/2 tsp baking soda
    1 tsp salt
    3 eggs

Directions

1. Place muffin cups in your 6-12 space tray.
2. Preheat oven to 350 degrees.
3. Blend yogurt, oil, vinegar, extract, and any sweetener you have together. Add the flour, salt, and baking soda. Blend until combined.
4. Now add in the eggs and blend again. Pop it on a high setting and blend for about 30 seconds until the eggs just mix in to create your batter.
5. Now add in all your other ingredients and stir by hand.
6. Place the batter into your muffin liners. Add some chopped walnuts or almonds on top if you wish.
7. Bake for around 15-20 minutes. To test if they're done, stick a knife or toothpick into the middle and see if it comes out clean. If not, then the muffins need to go back in for a few more minutes, just be sure to watch them carefully.

POPPY SEED MUFFINS

Ingredients:
- 3/4 cup almond flour
- 1/4 cup flaxseed meal
- 1/3 cup natural sweetener (Erythritol)
- 1tsp baking powder
- 1/4 cup unsalted butter
- 1/4 cup double cream
- 2 tbsp poppy seeds
- 3 eggs
- 3 tbsp lemon juice
- 1 tsp vanilla extract
- Natural sweetener to taste

Directions

1. Preheat the oven to 350.
2. Combine the flour, flaxseed, erythritol, and seeds
3. Melt the butter. Stir it into the flour with the cream and eggs. Create a smooth batter.
4. Add the rest of the ingredients.
5. Place 12 cupcake molds onto a baking tray and pour the mixture evenly into them. Silicone moulds are great for keeping the regular cost down.
6. Bake for around 20 minutes, until brown. You can also do the skewer test previously mentioned.
7. Allow to cool before serving.

PIZZA BREAKFAST FRITTATA

Ingredients:

   12 eggs
   9oz spinach or baby spinach
   1oz pepperoni
   1 tsp garlic, minced
   5oz mozzarella cheese
   1/2 cup ricotta cheese
   4 tbsp oil
   1/4 tsp nutmeg
   Seasoning to taste

Directions

1. Preheat the oven to 375.
2. Mix the eggs, spices, and oil together.
3. Add in the cheese and spinach.
4. Add to a skillet, sprinkle with some extra mozzarella cheese on top.
5. Add the pepperoni or any other desire toppings.
6. Place in the oven and bake for 30 minutes.

MOCK MCGRIDDLE LOAF

Ingredients
- 1 cup almond flour
- 1/4 cup flaxseed
- 1lb sausage
- 10 eggs
- 4oz cheese — cheddar or something similar
- 6 tbsp maple syrup
- 4 tbsp butter
- 1/2 tsp onion powder
- 1/2 tsp garlic powder
- 1/4 tsp sage
- Seasoning to taste

Directions
1. Pre-heat the oven to 350F degrees.
2. Add the sausage to a pan on the stove. Break up and cook until brown
3. Place all the dry ingredients into a bowl. Combine and add the wet ingredients, except for the 2 tbsp of maple syrup.
4. Add the sausage.
5. Place parchment paper into a casserole dish and add the mixture.
6. Drizzle the remaining syrup.
7. Bake for around 50 minutes, until completely cooked through.
8. Remove and allow to cool.

Try serving with some syrup or ketchup. It's perfect for that Sunday morning treat.

CAULIFLOWER AND JALAPENO CHEESE

*Ingredient*s for the puree:
  1 cauliflower head
  2 tbsp double cream
  1 tbsp butter
  1/4 cup cheese grated
  1 tbsp jalapenos, chopped
  1/4 tsp garlic powder
  Seasoning to taste

Ingredients for the cheese
  6 oz cream cheese
  1/2 cup cheese, shredded
  1/4 cup of salsa

*Ingredient*s for the topping
  3/4 cup Colby jack cheese, grated
  1/4 cup jalapenos, sliced

Directions
Puree
  1. Preheat the oven at 375.
  2. Break the cauliflower into medium sized pieces, then pop them in the microwave with the cream and butter for 10 minutes. Coat with the melted cream and butter and put in the microwave for another 6minutes.
  3. Remove and place in a blender with the rest of the ingredients. Blend until pureed.

Cream cheese:
1. Place the cream cheese in a bowl and microwave for 30 seconds.
2. Add the cheese and salsa, mixing completely.

Casserole Assembly
1. Spread the puree across a casserole dish.
2. Spread the cream cheese over the top.
3. Layer with your toppings.
4. Bake for 20 minutes.

If you choose to add vegetables, do so with the cream cheese layer.

KETO FRIENDLY SUSHI

Ingredients
- 16 oz cauliflower
- 6 oz softened cream cheese
- 2 tbsp rice vinegar
- 5 nori sheets
- 1 tbsp soy sauce
- 1 mini cucumber
- 2 avocados
- 5 oz of seafood of your choice

Directions

1. Grate the cauliflower.
2. Slice the ends of your cucumber off and then slice it in half, discarding the middle (seeds) of both. Then, slice into strips and set to one side.
3. Add cauliflower into a very hot pan, seasoning with soy sauce as it cooks.
4. Add the cauliflower to a bowl and mix in the cream cheese and vinegar. Set in the fridge to cool.
5. Once the rice is cooled, slice your avocado into small strips and remove the shell.
6. Place a nori sheet onto your bamboo roller. Spread on the rice, leaving about 3/4in at the top.
7. Place your fillers, layering just the way you want.
8. Roll the sushi with your bamboo roller. This will take some practice to get right.

Serve with wasabi and pickled ginger. You'll feel like you're in a Japanese restaurant, enjoying a local dish.

CHOCOLATE AND COCONUT BARS

Ingredients
- 1 cup unsweetened coconut, desiccated
- 1 packet natural sweetener (stevia)
- 1 tsp vanilla extract
- 1/3 cup coconut cream
- 4 tbsp coconut oil/cocoa butter
- 2 tbsp cocoa powder, unsweetened

Directions
1. Mix the coconut, cream, extract, and stevia together, mixing with a spoon.
2. Line a cookie sheet with parchment paper and place the coconut mixture on it.
3. Shape mixture into a rectangle, about 1in thick.
4. Freeze for two hours or until solid.
5. As you wait for it to cool, melt your coconut oil/cocoa butter in a sauce pan.
6. Add the powder, natural sweetner, and extract the oil. Mix and heat for 2 minutes.
7. Allow to cool until it is room temperature.
8. Remove the coconut from the freezer and cut into bars.
9. Dip the bars into the cocoa mixture, coating all sides evenly.
10. Place onto the cookie sheet and put into the fridge to cool completely.
11. Allow to remain in the fridge to keep the solid consistency when it comes to eating them.

If you want them softer, allow them to reaching room temperature.

CHOCOLATE MUG CAKE

Ingredients
  1 egg
  2 tbsp butter
  2 tbsp almond butter or protein powder
  2 tbsp cocoa powder, unsweetened
  1 1/2 tbsp Splenda
  2 tsp coconut flour
  1/4 tsp vanilla extract
  1/2 tsp baking powder

Directions
  1. Grab a mug and put 2tbsp of butter into it.
  2. Microwave for about 25 seconds until the butter hot and melted. Next, add the sweetener.
  3. Add the cocoa powder, coconut and almond flours, extract, baking powder, and egg.
  4. Mix until completely combined. You'll need to make sure there are no lumps for this to turn out just right.
  5. Microwave for about 75 seconds.

You can also make whip cream in a mixing bowl while making the cake, just remember to allow the cake to cool before you add the whipped cream on top!

CHOCOLATE AND PEANUT BUTTER TARTS

*Ingredient*s
Crust
    1/4 cup flaxseed ground until fine
    2 tbsp almond flour
    1 egg white
    1 tbsp sweetener

The middle layer:
    4 tbsp peanut butter (or nut butter of your choice)
    2 tbsp butter

The top layer:
    1 avocado
    4 tbsp cocoa powder, unsweetened
    1/4 cup sweetener
    1/2 tsp vanilla extract
    2 tbsp double cream
    1/2 cinnamon

Directions
1. Preheat the oven to 350F degrees.
2. Mix the ground flaxseeds and the rest of the crust ingredients until fully combined.
3. Press the mixture into a tart pan all the way up the sides.
4. Bake for 8 minutes until set.
5. Combine all the top layer ingredients in the blender. Smooth until creamy and set to one side.

6. Allow the crust to cool, while mixing your peanut butter and butter in the microwave.

7. Pour into the crust and refrigerate for 30 minutes until set.

8. Pour you top later over giving it a smooth texture and place in the fridge for an hour or so.

VEGAN POTATO NACHOS

Ingredients
- 3 cup potatoes, diced
- 1 jalapeno, thinly sliced
- 1 red pepper, finely chopped
- 1/2 cup pico de gallo
- 1 cup cooked black beans, (if canned, rinsed and drained)
- salt and pepper to taste
- 1/4 tsp garlic powder
- 2 Tbsp nutritional yeast
- 1 tsp chili powder
- 1/4 cup dairy-free milk (unsweetened almond milk)
- 1/2 orange pepper, roughly chopped
- 1/3 cup cashews, soaked at least two hours
- 1 tsp cumin
- 1 Tbsp olive oil
- Guacamole

Directions
Heat a cast iron pan to medium-high heat until it is very hot. Add oil and cook for 30 seconds then add potatoes and sprinkle with salt, pepper, and cumin. Cook, flipping occasionally, until crispy on all sides, about 15 minutes.

While the potatoes are cooking, make the cheese sauce. Place the cashews, orange pepper, milk, chili powder, nutritional yeast, garlic powder, and a pinch of salt/pepper in a blender. Puree until smooth, about 2-5 minutes depending on the blender being used. Blending for this long should make the cheese sauce hot, but if you want it hotter, you can heat up in the microwave or on the stove. Layer the nachos: potatoes, cheese sauce, black beans, pico de gallo, chopped red pepper, sliced jalapenos, and guacamole.

MUSHROOM AND KALE ENCHILADAS WITH RED SAUCE

Ingredients

2 tbsp olive oil

1/4 tsp ground black pepper

3 oz dried California chili pods, stems and seeds removed

1/3 cup yellow onion, chopped

2 garlic cloves

2 cup vegetable broth

1 tbsp dried chili powder

1 tsp dried cumin

1 tsp flour

1 tsp sugar

1/2 tsp salt

Directions

Place a skillet on medium heat. When hot, add the dried pepper pods and cook on each side for 20-30 seconds. Make sure they do not burn.

Remove from the skillet and add to a saucepan filled with hot water. Make sure the water covers the peppers. Let stand for 15 minutes, then drain.

While the peppers are in the water, add the oil to a skillet over medium heat. When hot, add the onion and cook for 3-4 minutes, followed by the garlic for 30 seconds or until fragrant.

Add the flour to the skillet and whisk. Add the chili powder, cumin, salt, black pepper, sugar, and vegetable broth. Mix well. Reduce to low heat.

Add the drained peppers and the mixture from the skillet into a blender. Blend until smooth. Note: depending on your blender, you may need to strain the mixture through a mesh strainer and discard the solid pieces.

ENCHILADAS

Ingredients
- 1/4 cup yellow onion, diced
- 2 garlic cloves, minced
- 8 oz cremini mushrooms, cleaned and diced
- 3 cup (packed) chopped kale
- 1/4 tsp salt
- 1/4 tsp ground black pepper
- 6 (8-inch) flour tortillas
- 2 oz Cotija cheese to sprinkle over the top
- Sour cream for garnish
- 2 tbsp olive oil
- Fresh cilantro leaves for garnish

Directions

Preheat the oven to 325F degrees.

Add the olive oil to a skillet over medium heat. When hot, add the onion and cook for 3-4 minutes, or until the onion begins to soften. Add the garlic and cook for 30 seconds before adding the mushrooms. Add the salt and black pepper and cook, stirring, until the mushrooms begin to release their juices. Add the kale and cook, stirring occasionally, until it softens. Remove from the heat and set aside.

Add the red sauce to a shallow skillet or bowl and place near the mushroom and kale mixture. Add 2 tbsps of the red sauce to the bottom of a 9x9-inch baking pan and spread it across the bottom. Place the pan next to the filling mixture.

One by one, dip each tortilla into the red sauce to cover both sides. Let the excess sauce drip back into the skillet. You may need to use your fingers to help remove some of the excess sauce. Lay each sauce-coated tortilla on a flat surface like a clean cutting board. Add about 2 heaping tbsps of the mushroom and kale mixture across the bottom edge of each tortilla, and leave a bit of room on either side, and at the bottom.

Starting with the end with the filling, roll the tortilla tightly to the other end. Then, place the rolled tortillas in the baking dish, seam side down. Pour about half of the remaining enchilada sauce over the rolled tortillas.

Cover with foil and bake for 30 minutes. Remove from the oven. Serve warm on individual plates with extra sauce on the side.

Drizzle with sour cream, and sprinkled with Cotija cheese and torn fresh cilantro.

SUPER EASY VEGGIE MAC AND CHEESE

Ingredients
   1 lb macaroni or other small noodle
   2 Tbsp butter
   2 Tbsp flour
   2 cup 2% milk
   2 cup shredded sharp cheddar cheese
   1 package Earthbound Farm frozen butternut squash, cooked and pureed until very smooth
   Salt and pepper to taste
   Optional: nutmeg

Directions
Cook pasta according to package *directions*.
Meanwhile, place butter in a large pot and heat over medium heat.
Once melted, sprinkle the flour on the butter and stir for 1-2 minutes.
Whisk in the milk, 1/2 cup at a time and cook until the flour has disappeared into the milk and the mixture has thickened, about 5 minutes, stirring constantly.
Stir in the pureed squash, then add the shredded cheese and continue to stir until mixture is smooth.
Season with salt, pepper, and nutmeg is desired.
When the pasta has finished cooking, drain and immediately mix into the cheese sauce.
Serve right away, with extra shredded cheese on top if desired.

WARM GREEN BEANS AND LETTUCE IN ANCHOVY BUTTER

Ingredients

- 4 Tbsp unsalted butter
- Chopped pistachios, for garnish
- 1 scallion, thinly sliced
- Pepper
- Sea salt
- 2 Tbsp fresh lemon juice, plus lemon wedges for serving
- 4 heads Little Gem or baby romaine lettuce, quartered lengthwise
- 2 garlic cloves, minced
- 6 oil-packed anchovy fillets, drained and chopped
- 1 lb green beans, trimmed
- Extra-virgin olive oil, for garnish

Directions

In a large skillet, melt 3 tbsps of the butter. Then, add the green beans, anchovies and garlic and cook over moderate heat, stirring occasionally, until the beans are tender, about 5 minutes. Transfer the beans to a large plate.

Add the remaining 1 tbsp of butter and the lettuce to the skillet and cook, turning occasionally, until the lettuce is golden and crisp-tender, about 2 minutes. Add the green beans and lemon juice and season with salt and pepper; toss to coat. Transfer the beans and lettuce to a serving platter and top with the sliced scallion. Top with pistachios, drizzle with olive oil and serve warm with lemon wedges

CONCLUSION

These recipes are a great way to get started with the vegetarian keto diet. They're not only fun and easy to make, but you'll barely notice the change. You'll be able to get your favourites like curries, sushi, pasta, and even sandwiches. With slight variations, you can cut out the carbs and focus on the fats that your body needs to create the ketones in the liver.

Go into this with full effort because you'll benefit from it in the end. Your mind will be in the zone, and you'll be able to enjoy a healthier lifestyle. Keep in mind that you're not saying "no" to anything, you're just finding ways to enjoy the things that you love without the things that are detrimental to your health.

Now that you've made the decision to follow the diet, it's time to choose the type.

When you want to add some carbs to a workout, you can follow the targeted ketogenic diet where you're allowed a few extra carbs, but only on the days and around the time of your workouts. After all, the focus is on still getting the exercise without struggling with energy. You wouldn't need to do this if you get enough fat into your diet and once your body gets into the ketone producing zone.

Now it's your turn – pick your diet and choose from the best vegeterian keto recipes for weight loss.

CPSIA information can be obtained
at www.ICGtesting.com
Printed in the USA
LVHW022335140121
676462LV00003B/535

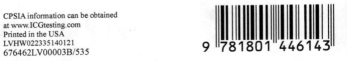